PERFECT WEIGHT LOSS TIPS

AN ULTIMATE GUIDE TO ACHIEVE WEIGHT LOSS PERFECT FOR YOUR SHAPE

MICHELLE TAYLOR

TABLE OF CONTENTS

INTRODUCTION

There was a time when our society didn't even think about losing weight. People ate what their mother made for dinner and went to work. The difference between this society and today's society was that work was done in fields and warehouses rather than behind computer screens. People worked physically because that was the only way to work. During this time, people were consuming far more calories than they burned, so they could eat whatever they wanted. But like all good things, it has come to an end, and technology in today's world has pushed us to be overweight. As the saying goes, every rose has a thorn, and in our society, the desire to live comfortably and work less begins to appear on the hips.

The bad thing about all of this is that the more weight you gain, the more dangerous it becomes. You need to lose weight to the point where you can't control yourself. It's not necessarily about getting toned and toned, it's about weight without being life-threatening. You can work on your abs later. For now, you just need to lose the excess body fat. As society realizes what's going on and that we're all overweight, people are trying to catch up. You can lose weight and lead a healthier lifestyle.

This eBook is your guide to losing that first 10 pounds that everyone struggles with. It's amazing how small life changes can lead to 10 pounds of weight loss, and they're all related to eating right and moving your body.

CHAPTER 1

WEIGHT LOSS STARTS WITH WHAT YOU DRINK

First of all, people don't realize that what they drink is the first step to losing their first 10 pounds. In fact, most people actually dehydrate when they're hungry unaware that it may be Also pay attention to water. Over 66% of our weight is water. This is another reason why water plays such an important role in weight management.

So tip 1 is: Drink lots of water. We recommend drinking 8 cups a day, but it can take some getting used to. Your body needs a lot of water. Not only does water wash away all toxins from your body, it also makes you feel better and healthier. The good thing about water is that it has zero calories, so you can drink as much as you like. Drinking lots of water will make you feel less hungry, so you will eat less. If you are hungry, try first a glass of water. You'll probably find yourself hydrated and not hungry at all. The key is to get the water your body needs.

Tip 2: Start your day with a clean glass of water. Drink immediately as soon as you wake up. A glass of water awakens all the digestive juices in the body and lubricates them well. You can drink coffee or tea anytime in the morning, but don't forget to drink a glass of water afterward. Caffeine dehydrates you and you want to keep dehydration at bay.

Tip 3: Drink a glass of water before you sit to eat. Water fills you up naturally, so you don't need to eat a lot.

Tip 4: Drink a glass of water with your meal. Taking each sip will help you feel full faster and leave the table feeling fuller.

Drinking water during a meal helps the food settle faster and makes you feel fuller sooner.

Tip 5: Avoid carbonated drinks as much as possible. All lemonades are sweetened with lots of sugar. The more you can eliminate from your diet, the better. Even diet soda is soda. It may not have a lot of sugar, but it also contains other chemicals and ingredients that are not good for you. If you drink soda, neutralize it with a glass of water. Remember that caffeine also dehydrates you. Decaffeinated sodas also contain as much sugar as a small amount of caffeine, making them not very healthy.

Tip 6: Fruit juices aren't as healthy as most people think. Juice actually contains a lot of sugar. When you crave a glass of juice, drink fresh fruit juice instead of artificially flavored or colored juices. Even better if you can make your own fruit juice. However, be careful not to add too much sugar as the calories will increase.

Tip 7: Limit your tea and coffee. As long as you don't add a lot of cream and sugar, it does little harm. It's cream and sugar that make you fat. Think of it this way. If you drink coffee or tea with cream and he has two sugar cubes, you're basically eating a slice of his chocolate cake every time. Think about how many slices of cake you eat while drinking a Venti Starbucks latte.

Tip 8: If you can give up alcohol, do it. Alcoholic drinks aren't good for you, but a glass of red wine is good for your heart, but mostly it just makes you fat. Beer makes you fat. Cocktails make you fat depending on their ingredients. For example whiskey and cola. Whiskey may not make you fat, but cola definitely does.

Tip 9: If you absolutely want alcohol, try dry wine. Dry wine is better than sweet wine because sweet wine has a lot of sugar. Dry wines contain sugars, most of which are fermented into alcohol, and dry wines are better in terms of weight gain.

Tip 10: A word about coffee. Not necessarily bad, but more interesting than anything else. Some people have found that drinking black coffee before exercise helps them lose weight. There is no scientific evidence for this, but nutritionists believe it may be because the body is forced to rely on fat for fuel. Hey, worth a try if you can stand black coffee. Remember to drink plenty of water while exercising!

Tip 11: Avoid drinking too much coffee as it desensitizes your body to the natural fat-burning effects of caffeine. 1-2 cups (if your day starts very slowly) max.

CHAPTER 2

EATING RIGHT AND LOSING WEIGHT

Now, when most people think of weight loss and diet, they think of diet. Unfortunately, all fad diets tend to make you fat. Why? They starve them to death until the man falls down and eats everything in sight. They also take away the food they love. This is neither a way to lose weight nor a way of life. You are actually only causing yourself stress that leads to weight gain! So when it comes to eating right, here are some tips that you can follow every day. Instead of depriving yourself of the foods you love, these tips will treat those foods as indulgences so you can enjoy them even more.

Tip 12: Eat fresh, juicy fruits and vegetables. These are foods such as tomatoes, watermelons, cantaloupe, kiwis and grapes. All of these fresh, flavorful, juicy fruits and vegetables are good for you. These foods are about 90-95% water, so you can eat more without gaining weight and still feel full.

Tip 13: Eat fresh fruits instead of processed fruits. Some are processed as more sugar. Processed, canned fruit also doesn't have as much fiber as fresh fruit.

Tip 14: Increase your fiber intake as much as possible. This usually means eating more fruits and vegetables.

Tip 15: Vegetables are your friend when it comes to weight loss. There are so many options here that you may want to try something you haven't tried before. Leafy green varieties are the best and I want you to work with salads as much as you can. They are packed with nutrients as long as you don't overdo it with dressing or add too much cheese. Leafy vegetables also contain plenty of natural water.

Tip 16: Watch what you eat. We don't just eat for the sake of eating. Animals eat instinctively. People eat when they know their body really needs it. Don't buy on impulse.

Tip 17: Be careful with everything you eat, from the food itself to the garnish. Garnishes and condiments are generally high in fat and can interfere with a healthy diet.

Tip 18: Be careful if you have a sweet tooth. That doesn't mean you can't eat sweets. Don't eat them as a meal. Always remember that these candies add to areas you don't want to add to. But don't go without it.

Tip 19: Set meal times and stick to them. Have your meals at specific times and try to eat at those times. Eating habits help you control what and when you eat. Also, eating 5 small meals a day is much better than 1 or 2 large meals. Also, don't wait until you're hungry. This will make you overeat until you are full.

Tip 20: Eat only when you're hungry. Drink a glass of water first to determine if you are really hungry or thirsty. Most people tend to eat when they see food. That doesn't mean they're hungry. They just want to eat it. Don't eat anything offered to you unless you're really hungry. If you want to eat it as a courtesy, just take a bite and don't eat it.

Tip 21: Don't snack between meals, but if you must, make sure it's a healthy snack. If you travel a lot, look for healthy snacks instead of junk food.

Tip 22: Vegetables make great snacks. They can get you through hunger pangs if you have them. Carrots are great because they satisfy hunger and are packed with nutrients.

Tip 23: For those who need groceries, it's a good idea to count calories. For processed foods, the calorie count is displayed on the package. Be careful with your serving

Tip 24: Avoid fried foods. If you want bread crumbs, it's better to bake. Fried foods are dipped in oil and eaten. Even after the excess oil has been drained, the oil is still absorbed by the food itself.

Tip 25: Don’t skip meals. It is recommended that you eat at least 3 small meals a day, preferably 5. This will prevent you from feeling hungry or overeating due to hunger during the day.

Tip 26: You should only eat one egg a day. If you can reduce your egg intake to 3 per week, that’s great.

Tip 27: Chocolate should be treated as a luxury item. Buy good food and eat it only occasionally. Savoring every bite doubles the joy of eating and doubles the deliciousness.

Tip 28: Eat foods from all food groups every day. This is a great way to make sure your body gets all the nutrients it needs and help prevent nutritional deficiencies. Experiment so you don’t get bored with the same old diet.

Tip 29: Eat breakfast within an hour of waking up. This is the best way to give your body the jump start it needs. Don’t wait until you're really hungry. Breakfast is important, but it doesn't have to fill you up. The idea is to break the fast because you haven't eaten all night.

CHAPTER 3

CHANGE YOUR DIET TO LOSE WEIGHT

Here are some tips to help you lose your first 10 pounds by simply changing the way you prepare your meals. How a food is prepared has as much to do with how healthy it is.

Tip 30: Try baking these things instead of frying them in oil or oil. Baking does not require all of the fats and oils required for frying, nor does food become saturated with these substances during cooking.

Tip 31: Use a non-stick pan spray to avoid oil. Also, a non-stick frying pan doesn't need much oil, even if it does.

Tip 32: Cook vegetables instead of boiling them. You can also steam foods such as cabbage, cauliflower, broccoli, and carrots, as this is probably the healthiest way to eat them.

Tip 33: Be careful with fat-free and low-fat foods. There are many of these foods on the market, but they are not necessarily healthy. Many of these foods are sweetened with some type of chemical or carbohydrate to improve their taste. However, the body converts these chemicals and carbohydrates into sugars within the body. That is, they are still converted into fat.

Tip 34: Don't fall victim to crash diets. These things are bad for you and will end up doing more harm than good in the long run. , the second time the weight is worse. You won't survive on crash diets and it's time to quit.

CHAPTER 4

EXERCISE TO LOSE WEIGHT

There are two things you need to do to lose weight, and you already know one. This means eating right and filling your body with good, clean water. Another thing you need is to move your body. You don't have to buy a gym membership to work out. In fact, there are some things you can do on a daily basis to lose weight. There are also some exercises you can do yourself to lose weight.

Tip 35: Once you start exercising, whether at home or in the gym, don't be discouraged if you don't see immediate results. It takes a week or more to get your body in shape and make progress. Many people assume that a workout doesn't work if it takes a little longer.

Putting too much stress on your body when you start exercising can lead to injury. Your bones, joints and ligaments are not ready for the stress you put on them. Unfortunately, that's not how the body works. When it comes to training, slow and steady win the race.

Tip 36: Check your weight when you start exercising, but don't use it as a guide to weight loss. Weight fluctuates throughout the day. Checking your weight every day may only discourage you.

Tip 37: The best way to tell if you're losing weight is how your clothes fit. When you feel like you're floating in your clothes, you know that diet and exercise are good for you. Another way you can tell if you're losing weight is if you can move where you normally wear your belt.

Tip 38: Checking your weight and the fit of your clothes regularly pays off. Buy new running shoes or new jeans. This will help you stay motivated as you pursue your weight loss goals.

Tip 39: Take a day off from exercise to give your body a chance to rest and repair. Once a week, the body needs a rest day.

Tip 40: Three days of 30-minute workouts can help you maintain your weight, but you needs at least four days of 30-minute workouts to start losing weight. Five days a week is even more effective.

Tip 41: Gather information about exercises and simple things you can do at home. There is a wealth of research on exercise, allowing you to choose the one that will help you reach your weight loss goals the most. Surf the internet or pick up some health and exercise books at your local bookstore or library to learn how to burn the number of calories you're trying to burn each week.

Tip 42: Try finding a training partner. This must be someone who is as committed to exercise and weight loss as you are. One of the benefits of finding a committed partner is that he feels accountable to his partner. It means that there are people. Knowing that someone is waiting for you makes it easier to get up and work out together. You don't want to wake your workout partner, do you?

Tip 43: When your body says it's enough, take a break. When you exercise for a long time, your body starts sending signals. This is especially important if you are just starting an exercise intensity

Tip 44: If you increase the length of your workouts, do so gradually. The same applies to training intensity.

Tip 45: Choose an exercise routine that fits your lifestyle. Everyone has a different lifestyle and does a different job.

There is no set time when you should or shouldn't exercise. It's relaxing, so if you like working out late before bed, do it. If you like working out early in the morning because it helps you wake up, that's great too. Some people like to exercise to recover from work stress or during their lunch break.

Tip 46: Walk around instead of standing. If you can walk around, do it. People with pacemakers are actually doing a lot because they are constantly moving. Pacing also helps thinking.

Tip 47: If you can stand, don't sit. Standing comfortably burns more calories than sitting.

Tip 48: If you can sit, don't lie down.

Tip 49: Couches and TVs can help you lose weight. If you tend to be a couch potato, don't sit. If unavoidable, put an uncomfortable chair in front of the TV and avoid spending too much time in front of it. The same applies to computers.

If you are a computer junkie. Some people put their chairs in front of the computer more than in front of the TV. (Of course, this applies if you have to work long hours in front of a computer, not telecommuting, as a chair becomes very important in such cases.)

Tip 50: If you have a sedentary job, get up and stretch every 30 minutes. Most of today's work is done in front of a computer and requires sitting down. If you have a job like this, you have to move once in a while.

Tip 51: During commercial breaks, walk around, do simple exercises like crunches, Bend down and touch your toes. Do whatever it takes to get your body moving and your blood pumping.

Tip 52: Turn on music and dance. Again, the more you exercise, the better you feel and the more weight you lose.

Tip 53: If you're taking public transit, get off one block before the stop and walk the rest of the way. This is a great way to plan a walk before or after work or on your way to another destination.

Tip 54: Twist your pelvis to tone your core. Of course, you won't be doing these with anyone else around you, but they're a good step to prepare your body for more serious exercise.

Stomach cramps. It also works on the muscles in your back, allowing you to relax without feeling tight.

Tip 55: Lift weights. Strength training burns more fat than you believe. When you work on building muscle, you start burning fat to promote muscle growth. When building muscle, keep in mind that muscle weighs more than fat, so a scale is not an accurate tool for determining weight loss.

Tip 56: Massage your partner. They can put in a little effort and at the same time make up for the weight they've lost if they're training with you. Tip 86: Always use two stairs, not just one. This will make you work harder and increase your heart rate.

CHAPTER 5

GETTING STARTED

Now that you know how to get started, let's talk a little bit more about weight loss and weight loss. It all starts with what you eat. We are fatter than ever, so fat and weight loss are very important aspects of our lives today. Increase. In fact, it is one of the most popular keywords people search on the internet today.

The main reason we are overweight is because of our relationship with food. We tend to focus on quantity. We want as much as we can get, not the best food we can get. Quantity always trumps quality when it should be the exact opposite.

Once you've decided to lose weight, it can be difficult to know exactly where to start. If you have the determination to build momentum and lose weight, it is possible. You have to understand how to say "no".

Everyone is different. No one else has the same metabolism as you or burns fat like you do. You may be the exact same weight as the person next to you, but if you both start an exercise and diet program, even if you do the exact same thing to everyone, two weeks later or he's the same weight in a month. You may not get any results. It's important to know that not everyone uses food in the same way. What one person gains weight may not be the same for another. The same applies to weight loss. Let's say you're a married woman and you and your husband work out together and he stopped drinking soda and lost 5 pounds. Because he stopped drinking soda. Eating and exercising exactly the same won't necessarily give you the same results.

The bottom line is that today's society has to work much harder than the societies of the past. Sixty years ago, women and men were thin because they had to work. Manual labor was required. Otherwise there was nothing to eat. Eggs had to be obtained from chicken coops when they were wanted, cows had to be milked to get fresh milk, and fields had to be plowed to grow vegetables. If you wanted beef, you had to know a little bit about fattening and slaughtering veal. That was life back then, and technology has removed all that manual work. Instead, you should watch what you eat and move. Otherwise there is little reason to move.

It's very important to understand that weight loss goals can vary greatly depending on how hard you work. The only thing in life that requires manual labor

Achieve if you want to see results. Generally, you don't have to worry about losing weight until you're in your 20s, but with today's fast food lifestyle, that's not always the case. When you're shopping for groceries for you and your family, read the ingredients of what you're eating. If you can't pronounce it, don't eat it. Processed foods trigger appetite, and appetite leads to weight gain. This is especially important if you want to lose and maintain weight.

However, you can't lose weight just by watching your diet. Proper nutrition should also be combined with the right amount of exercise. The solution is a training regiment

Give your body the exercise it needs to burn fat and calories efficiently. It's almost like hibernating when it's not moving, especially when it just gains weight around it.

CONSTISTENCY IS KEY

Consistency is the most important aspect of any training program. If you have a goal, you can definitely achieve it if you keep working towards it.

Getting started is usually easy for people. Go shopping, buy workout clothes, shop running shoes and a gym membership. After that, they go to training fairly consistently for a week or two. However, as time goes on, they find it difficult to maintain a routine. Life is getting tougher and they go to the gym less and less. In other words, their gym membership is gone and they just stop going.

Many people choose to exercise in the evening, but for some this routine is even more difficult. If you don't come home from work completely exhausted, this is the one for you.

Good time. But if you can't do that, you may need to find a way to get there

Morning. It can help you stay awake and maintain your consistency.

There is a misconception that exercise makes you tired, but that is not always the case. You may feel like this for the first few times, but as you get in better shape, you will find that you have more energy. Plus, you'll feel energized throughout the day, so you'll feel better throughout the day.

Even if you don't have a gym membership, chances are that some people have sidewalks in front of their homes and access to the pool. Let's play sports. If you have four-legged friends, I'm sure they'll have fun with you too.

www.ingramcontent.com/pod-product-compliance
Lightning Source LLC
LaVergne TN
LVHW020542160826
845677LV00015B/4163

* 9 7 9 8 3 5 1 7 0 0 4 5 8 *